The Ultimate Air Fryer Seafood Cooking Guide

Healthy Air Fryer Seafood Recipes To Lose Weight

Ellie Sloan

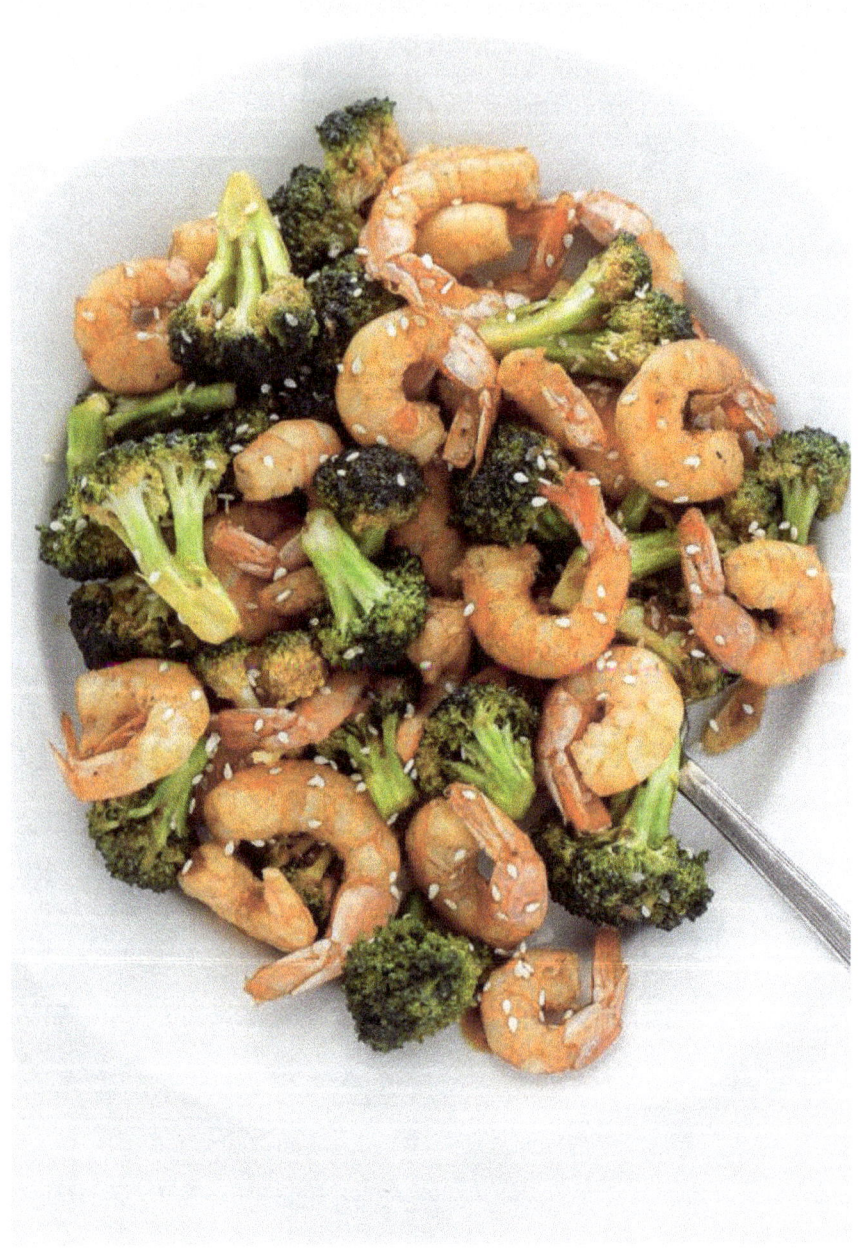

© Copyright 2020 - All rights reserved.

The content contained within this book may not be reproduced, duplicated or transmitted without direct written permission from the author or the publisher.

Under no circumstances will any blame or legal responsibility be held against the publisher, or author, for any damages, reparation, or monetary loss due to the information contained within this book. Either directly or indirectly.

Legal Notice:

This book is copyright protected. This book is only for personal use. You cannot amend, distribute, sell, use, quote or paraphrase any part, or the content within this book, without the consent of the author or publisher.

Disclaimer Notice:

Please note the information contained within this document is for educational and entertainment purposes only. All effort has been executed to present accurate, up to date, and reliable, complete information. No warranties of any kind are declared or implied. Readers acknowledge that the author is not engaging in the rendering of legal, financial, medical or professional advice. The content within this book has been derived from various sources. Please consult a licensed professional before attempting any techniques outlined in this book.

By reading this document, the reader agrees that under no circumstances is the author responsible for any losses, direct or indirect, which are incurred as a result of the use of information contained within this document, including, but not limited to, — errors, omissions, or inaccuracies.

Table of contents

Grilled Beetroots and Broccolini. **Errore. Il segnalibro non è definito.**

Grilled Artichokes and Mustard Greens**Errore. Il segnalibro non è definito.**

Grilled Beets and Swiss Chard .... **Errore. Il segnalibro non è definito.**

Grilled Baby Corn and Winter Squash**Errore. Il segnalibro non è definito.**

Grilled Beets and Asparagus .... **Errore. Il segnalibro non è definito.**

Grilled Artichoke.......................... **Errore. Il segnalibro non è definito.**

Grilled Summer Squash Cabbage and Romaine Lettuce**Errore. Il segnalibro non è definito.**

Grilled Rutabaga Baby Carrots and Brussels Sprouts**Errore. Il segnalibro non è definito.**

Grilled Kale Beets and Carrots.... **Errore. Il segnalibro non è definito.**

Grilled Turnip Greens Okra and Red Onion**Errore. Il segnalibro non è definito.**

Grilled Collard Greens Artichoke , Carrots and Kale**Errore. Il segnalibro non è definito.**

Grilled Water Chestnuts and Asparagus**Errore. Il segnalibro non è definito.**

Grilled Butternut Squash with Chipotle**Errore. Il segnalibro non è definito.**

Grilled Beetroots with Poblano Chilies**Errore. Il segnalibro non è definito.**

Grilled Portbello Mushrooms with Almond Lemon Dip**Errore. Il segnalibro non è definito.**

Grilled Smoky Butternut Squash with Vegan Yogurt**Errore. Il segnalibro non è definito.**

Grilled Cauliflower Broccoli and Asparagus**Errore. Il segnalibro non è definito.**

Grilled Spiraled Eggplants with Tomatoes**Errore. Il segnalibro non è definito.**

Shishito Peppers Skewers With Teriyaki Glaze Recipe**Errore. Il segnalibro non è definito.**

Avocado Lima Beans and Tomato Bowl**Errore. Il segnalibro non è definito.**

Brussels Tempeh with Soy Dressing**Errore. Il segnalibro non è definito.**

Vegetarian Creamy Spaghetti Carbonara**Errore. Il segnalibro non è definito.**

Quinoa with Pesto Cream .... **Errore. Il segnalibro non è definito.**

Southeast Asian Fried Rice .... **Errore. Il segnalibro non è definito.**

Vegetarian Spaghetti .... **Errore. Il segnalibro non è definito.**

Curried Lima Beans .... **Errore. Il segnalibro non è definito.**

Kale and Quorn Pesto Salad .... **Errore. Il segnalibro non è definito.**

Vegetarian Tofu Wrap .... **Errore. Il segnalibro non è definito.**

Vegetarian Navy Bean Chili .... **Errore. Il segnalibro non è definito.**

Lima Bean and Pea Salad .... **Errore. Il segnalibro non è definito.**

Broccoli & Basmati Rice Pilaf ...... **Errore. Il segnalibro non è definito.**

Avocado Pasta .... **Errore. Il segnalibro non è definito.**

Vegetarian Quorn Salad .... **Errore. Il segnalibro non è definito.**

Mexican Spaghettini Soup........... **Errore. Il segnalibro non è definito.**

Blueberry and Kale Citrus Salad . **Errore. Il segnalibro non è definito.**

Spinach Stir Fry .... **Errore. Il segnalibro non è definito.**

Easy Kale Stir Fry .... **Errore. Il segnalibro non è definito.**

Choy Sum Stir Fry........................ **Errore. Il segnalibro non è definito.**

Vegetarian Stuffed Crust Pizza.... **Errore. Il segnalibro non è definito.**

Avocado and Lima Bean Salad Sandwich**Errore. Il segnalibro non è definito.**

Roasted Cauliflower and Garbanzo Beans**Errore. Il segnalibro non è definito.**

Roasted Tomato Broccoli and Chickpeas**Errore. Il segnalibro non è definito.**

Roasted Soybean and Broccoli.... **Errore. Il segnalibro non è definito.**

Buttery Roasted Tomatoes and Edamame Beans**Errore. Il segnalibro non è definito.**

Roasted Choy Sum and Button Mushroom**Errore. Il segnalibro non è definito.**

Simple Roasted Mustard Greens **Errore. Il segnalibro non è definito.**

Roasted Mustard Greens and Red Cabbage Extra**Errore. Il segnalibro non è definito.**

Roasted Spinach and Artichoke Hearts Extra**Errore. Il segnalibro non è definito.**

Roasted Parsnips and Watercress Extra**Errore. Il segnalibro non è definito.**

Roasted Napa Cabbage Baby Carrots and Watercress Extra**Errore. Il segnalibro non è definito.**

Roasted Artichoke Hearts and Napa Cabbage Extra**Errore. Il segnalibro non è definito.**

Char-Grilled Spicy Halibut

Preparation Time: 5 minutes

Cooking Time: 20 minutes

Servings: 4

Ingredients:

- 3 lb. halibut fillet, skin removed
- Salt and pepper to taste
- 4 tbsp. olive oil
- 2 cloves of garlic, minced
- 1 tbsp. chili powder

Directions:

1. Place all ingredients in a Ziploc bag.
2. Keep it in the fridge for at least 2 hours.
3. Preheat the Air Fryer at 390°F.
4. Place the grill pan attachment in the Air Fryer.
5. Grill the fish for 20 minutes while flipping every 5 minutes.

Nutrition:

Calories 385

Fat 40.6g

Carbs 1.7g

Protein 33g

Swordfish with Charred Leeks

Preparation Time: 5 minutes

Cooking Time: 20 minutes

Servings: 4

Ingredients:

- 4 swordfish steaks
- Salt and pepper to taste
- 3 tbsp. lime juice
- 2 tbsp. olive oil
- 4 medium leeks, cut into an inch long

Directions:

1. Preheat the Air Fryer at 390°F. Place the grill pan attachment in the Air Fryer.
2. Season the swordfish with salt, pepper and lime juice.
3. Brush the fish with olive oil. Place fish fillets on grill pan and top with leeks.
4. Grill for 20 minutes.

Nutrition:

Calories 611

Fat 40g

Carbs 14.6g

Protein 48g

Breaded Coconut Shrimp

Preparation Time: 5 minutes

Cooking Time: 15 minutes

Servings: 4

Ingredients:

- Shrimp (1 lb.)
- Panko breadcrumbs (1 cup)
- Shredded coconut (1 cup)
- Eggs (2)
- All-purpose flour (.33 cup)

Directions:

1. Fix the temperature of the Air Fryer at 360°F.
2. Peel and devein the shrimp.
3. Whisk the seasonings with the flour as desired. In another dish, whisk the eggs, and in the third container, combine the breadcrumbs and coconut.

4. Dip the cleaned shrimp into the flour, egg wash, and finish it off with the coconut mixture.
5. Lightly spray the basket of the fryer and set the timer for 10-15 minutes.
6. Air-fry until it's a golden brown before serving.

Nutrition:

Calories 285

Fat 12.8g

Carbs 3.7g

Protein 38.1g

Breaded Cod Sticks

Preparation Time: 5 minutes

Cooking Time: 20 minutes

Servings: 4

Ingredients:

- Large eggs (2)
- Milk (3 tbsp.)
- Breadcrumbs (2 cups)
- Almond flour (1 cup)
- Cod (1 lb.)

Directions:

1. Heat the Air Fryer at 350°F.
2. Prepare three bowls; one with the milk and eggs, one with the breadcrumbs (salt and pepper if desired), and another with almond flour.
3. Dip the sticks in the flour, egg mixture, and breadcrumbs.

4. Place in the basket and set the timer for 12 minutes. Toss the basket halfway through the cooking process.
5. Serve with your favorite sauce.

Nutrition:

Calories 254

Fat 14.2g

Carbs 5.7g

Protein 39.1g

Cajun Salmon

Preparation Time: 5 minutes

Cooking Time: 10 minutes

Servings: 2

Ingredients:

- Salmon fillet (1 - 7 oz.) 0.75-inches thick
- Cajun seasoning
- Juice (¼ of a lemon)
- Optional: Sprinkle of sugar

Directions:

1. Set the Air Fryer at 356°F to preheat for five minutes.
2. Rinse and dry the salmon with a paper towel. Cover the fish with the Cajun coating mix.
3. Place the fillet in the Air Fryer for seven minutes with the skin side up.
4. Serve with a sprinkle of lemon and dusting of sugar if desired.

Nutrition:

Calories 285

Fat 17.8g

Carbs 6.8g

Protein 42.1g

Cajun Shrimp

Preparation Time: 5 minutes

Cooking Time: 5 minutes

Servings: 6

Ingredients:

- Tiger shrimp (16-20/1.25 lb.)
- Olive oil (1 tbsp.)
- Old Bay seasoning (.5 tsp.)
- Smoked paprika (.25 tsp.)
- Cayenne pepper (.25 tsp.)

Directions:

1. Set the Air Fryer at 390°F.
2. Cover the shrimp using the oil and spices.
3. Toss them into the Air Fryer basket and set the timer for five minutes.
4. Serve with your favorite side dish.

Nutrition:

Calories 356

Fat 18g

Carbs 5g

Protein 34g

Codfish Nuggets

Preparation Time: 5 minutes

Cooking Time: 20 minutes

Servings: 4

Ingredients:

- Cod fillet (1 lb.)
- Eggs (3)
- Olive oil (4 tbsp.)
- Almond flour (1 cup)
- Gluten-free breadcrumbs (1 cup)

Directions:

1. Warm the Air Fryer at 390°F.
2. Slice the cod into nuggets.
3. Prepare three bowls. Whisk the eggs in one. Combine the salt, oil, and breadcrumbs in another. Sift the almond flour into the third one.

4. Cover each of the nuggets with the flour, dip in the eggs, and the breadcrumbs.
5. Arrange the nuggets in the basket and set the timer for 20 minutes.
6. Serve the fish with your favorite dips or sides.

Nutrition:

Calories 334

Fat 10g

Carbs 8g

Protein 32g

Creamy Salmon

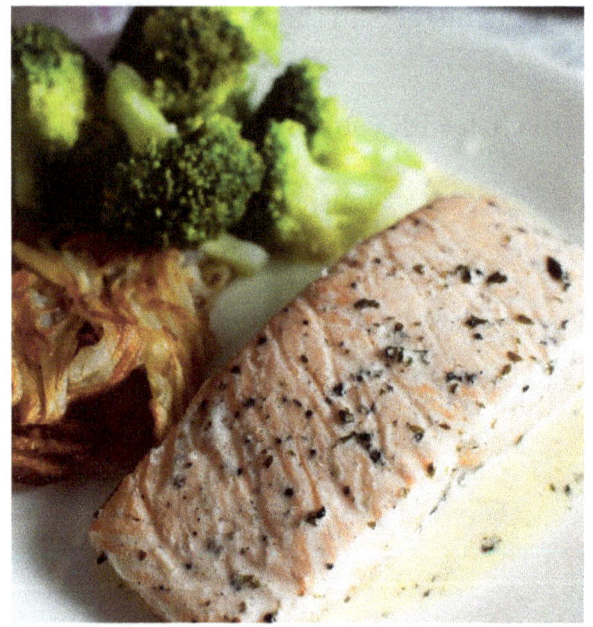

Preparation Time: 5 minutes

Cooking Time: 20 minutes

Servings: 4

Ingredients:

- Chopped dill (1 tbsp.)

- Olive oil (1 tbsp.)
- Sour cream (3 tbsp.)
- Plain yogurt (1.76 oz.)
- Salmon (6 pieces)/.75 lb.)

Directions:

1. Heat the Air Fryer and wait for it to reach 285°F.
2. Shake the salt over the salmon and add them to the fryer basket with the olive oil to air-fry for 10 minutes.
3. Whisk the yogurt, salt, and dill.
4. Serve the salmon with the sauce with your favorite sides.

Nutrition:

Calories 340

Carbs 5g

Fat 16g

Protein 32g

Crumbled Fish

Preparation Time: 5 minutes

Cooking Time: 15 minutes

Servings: 4

Ingredients:

- Breadcrumbs (.5 cup)
- Vegetable oil (4 tbsp.)
- Egg (1)
- Fish fillets (4)
- Lemon (1)

Directions:

1. Heat the Air Fryer to reach 356°F.
2. Whisk the oil and breadcrumbs until crumbly.
3. Dip the fish into the egg, then the crumb mixture.
4. Arrange the fish in the cooker and air-fry for 12 minutes.
5. Garnish using the lemon.

Nutrition:

Calories 320

Carbs 8g

Fat 10g

Protein 28g

Easy Crab Sticks

Preparation Time: 5 minutes

Cooking Time: 10 minutes

Servings: 4

Ingredients:

- Crab sticks (1 package)
- Cooking oil spray (as needed)

Directions:

1. Take each of the sticks out of the package and unroll it until the stick is flat. Tear the sheets into thirds.
2. Arrange them on the Air Fryer basket and lightly spritz using cooking spray. Set the timer for 10 minutes at 360°F.
3. Note: If you shred the crab meat, you can cut the time in half, but they will also easily fall through the holes in the basket.

Nutrition:

Calories 285

Fat 12.8g

Carbs 3.7g

Protein 38.1g

Fried Catfish

Preparation Time: 5 minutes

Cooking Time: 15 minutes

Servings: 4

Ingredients:

- Olive oil (1 tbsp.)
- Seasoned fish fry (.25 cup)
- Catfish fillets (4)

Directions:

1. Heat the Air Fryer to reach 400°F before fry time.
2. Rinse the catfish and pat dry using a paper towel.
3. Dump the seasoning into a sizeable zipper-type bag. Add the fish and shake to cover each fillet. Spray with a spritz of cooking oil spray and add to the basket.
4. Set the timer for 10 minutes. Flip and reset the timer for ten additional minutes. Turn the fish once more and cook for 2-3 minutes.

5. Once it reaches the desired crispiness, transfer to a plate, and serve.

Nutrition:

Calories 376

Fat 9g

Carbs 10g

Protein 28g

Grilled Sardines

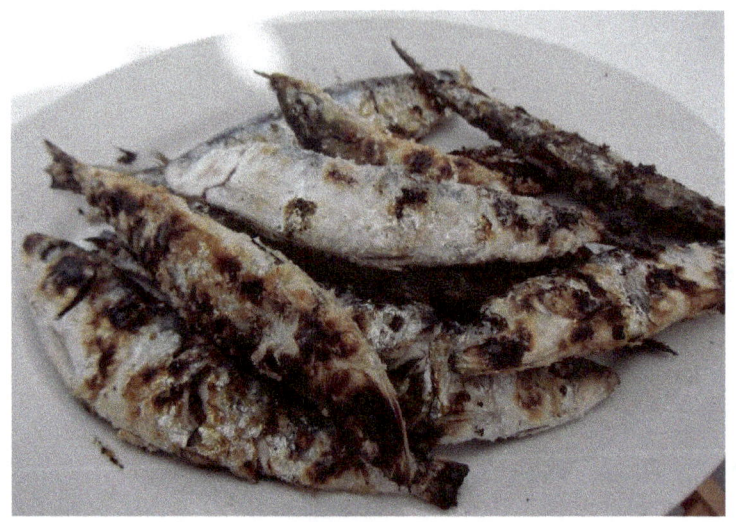

Preparation Time: 5 minutes

Cooking Time: 20 minutes

Servings: 4

Ingredients:

- 5 sardines
- Herbs of Provence

Directions:

1. Preheat the Air Fryer to 320°F.
2. Spray the basket and place your sardines in the basket of your fryer.
3. Set the timer for 14 minutes. After 7 minutes, remember to turn the sardines so that they are roasted on both sides.

Nutrition:

Calories 189

Fat 10g

Carbs 0g

Protein 22g

Zucchini with Tuna

Preparation Time: 10 minutes

Cooking Time: 30 minutes

Servings: 4

Ingredients:

- 4 medium zucchinis
- 4 oz. of tuna in oil (canned) drained
- 1 oz. grated cheese
- 1 tsp. pine nuts
- Salt, pepper to taste

Directions:

1. Cut the zucchini in half laterally and empty it with a small spoon (set aside the pulp that will be used for the filling); place them in the basket.
2. In a food processor, put the zucchini pulp, drained tuna, pine nuts and grated cheese. Mix everything until you get a homogeneous and dense mixture.

3. Fill the zucchini. Set the Air Fryer to 360°F.
4. Air fry for 20 min. depending on the size of the zucchini. Let cool before serving

Nutrition:

Calories 389

Carbs 10g

Fat 29g

Protein 23g

Caramelized Salmon Fillet

Preparation Time: 5 minutes

Cooking Time: 25 minutes

Servings: 4

Ingredients:

- 2 salmon fillets
- 2 oz. cane sugar
- 4 tbsp. soy sauce
- 1.7 oz. sesame seeds
- Unlimited Ginger

Directions:

1. Preheat the Air Fryer at 360°F for 5 minutes.
2. Put the sugar and soy sauce in the basket. Cook everything for 5 minutes.
3. In the meantime, wash the fish well, pass it through sesame to cover it completely and place it inside the tank and add the fresh ginger.

4. Cook for 12 minutes. Turn the fish over and finish cooking for another 8 minutes.

Nutrition:

Calories 569

Fat 14.9g

Carbs 40g

Protein 66.9g

Deep Fried Prawns

Preparation Time: 15 minutes

Cooking Time: 10 minutes

Servings: 6

Ingredients:

- 12 prawns
- 2 eggs
- Flour to taste
- Breadcrumbs
- 1 tsp. oil

Directions:

1. Remove the head of the prawns and shell carefully.
2. Pass the prawns first in the flour, then in the beaten egg and then in the breadcrumbs.
3. Preheat the Air Fryer for 1 minute at 300°F.
4. Add the prawns and cook for 4 minutes. If the prawns are large, it will be necessary to cook 6 at a time.

5. Turn the prawns and cook for another 4 minutes.
6. They should be served with a yogurt or mayonnaise sauce.

Nutrition:

Calories 2385

Fat 23g

Carbs 52.3g

Protein 21.4g

Mussels with Pepper

Preparation Time: 15 minutes

Cooking Time: 12 minutes

Servings: 5

Ingredients:

- 25 oz. mussels
- 1 clove garlic
- 1 tsp. oil
- Pepper to taste
- Parsley Taste

Directions:

1. Clean and scrape the mold cover and remove the byssus (the "beard" that comes out of the mold).
2. Pour the oil, clean the mussels and the crushed garlic in the Air Fryer basket. Set the temperature to 390°F and simmer for 12 minutes. Towards the end of cooking, add black pepper and chopped parsley.

3. Finally, distribute the mussel juice well at the bottom of the basket, stirring the basket.

Nutrition:

Calories 150

Carbs 2g

Fat 8g

Protein 15g

Monkfish with Olives and Capers

Preparation Time: 25 minutes

Cooking Time: 40 minutes

Servings: 4

Ingredients:

- 1 monkfish
- 10 cherry tomatoes
- 1.75 oz. cailletier olives
- 5 capers

Directions:

1. Spread aluminum foil inside the Air Fryer basket and place the monkfish clean and skinless.
2. Add chopped tomatoes, olives, capers, oil, and salt.
3. Set the temperature to 320°F.
4. Cook the monkfish for about 40 minutes.

Nutrition:

Calories 404

Fat 29g

Carbs 36g

Protein 24g

Shrimp, Zucchini and Cherry Tomato Sauce

Preparation Time: 5 minutes

Cooking Time: 25 minutes

Servings: 4

Ingredients:

- 2 zucchinis
- 10 oz. shrimp
- 7 cherry tomatoes
- Salt and pepper to taste
- 1 clove garlic

Directions:

1. Pour the oil in the Air Fryer, add the garlic clove and diced zucchini.
2. Cook for 15 minutes at 300°F. Add the shrimps and the pieces of tomato, salt, and spices.

3. Cook for another 5 to 10 minutes or until the shrimp water evaporates.

Nutrition:

Calories 214.3

Fat 8.6g

Carbs 7.8g

Protein 27.0g

Salmon with Pistachio Bark

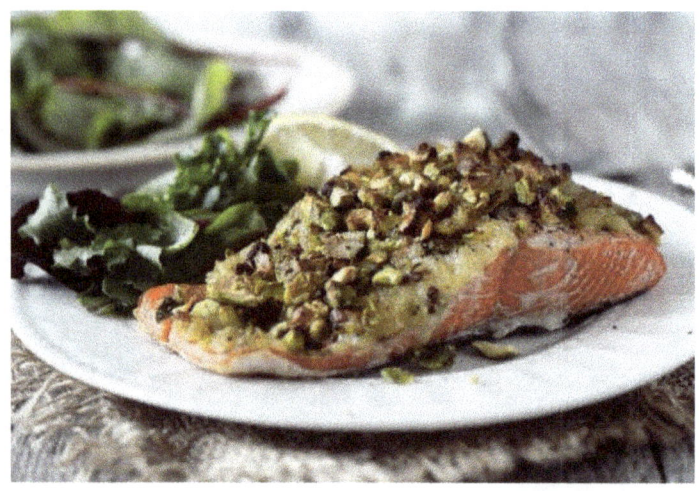

Preparation Time: 10 minutes

Cooking Time: 30 minutes

Servings: 4

Ingredients:

- 20 oz. salmon fillet
- 1.75 oz. pistachios
- Salt to taste

Directions:

1. Put the parchment paper on the bottom of the Air Fryer basket and place the salmon fillet in it (it can be cooked whole or already divided into four portions).
2. Cut the pistachios in thick pieces; grease the top of the fish, salt (little because the pistachios are already salted) and cover everything with the pistachios.
3. Set the Air Fryer to 360°F and simmer for 25 minutes.

Nutrition:

Calories 371.7

Fat 21.8g

Carbs 9.4g

Protein 34.7g

Salted Marinated Salmon

Preparation Time: 10 minutes

Cooking Time: 30 minutes

Servings: 4

Ingredients:

- 17 oz. salmon fillet
- 2 lb. coarse salt

Directions:

1. Place the baking paper on the Air Fryer basket and the salmon on top (skin side up) covered with coarse salt.
2. Set the Air Fryer to 300°F.
3. Cook everything for 25 to 30 minutes. At the end of cooking, remove the salt from the fish and serve with a drizzle of oil.

Nutrition:

Calories 290

Fat 13g

Carbs 3g

Protein 40g

Sautéed Trout with Almonds

Preparation Time: 35 minutes

Cooking Time: 20 minutes

Servings: 4

Ingredients:

- 25 oz. salmon trout
- 15 black peppercorns
- Dill leaves to taste
- 1 oz. almonds
- Salt to taste

Directions:

1. Cut the trout into cubes and marinate it for half an hour with the rest of the ingredients (except salt).
2. Cook in Air Fryer for 17 minutes at 320°F. Pour a drizzle of oil and serve.

Nutrition:

Calories 238.5

Fat 20.1g

Carbs 11.5g

Protein4.0g

Rabas

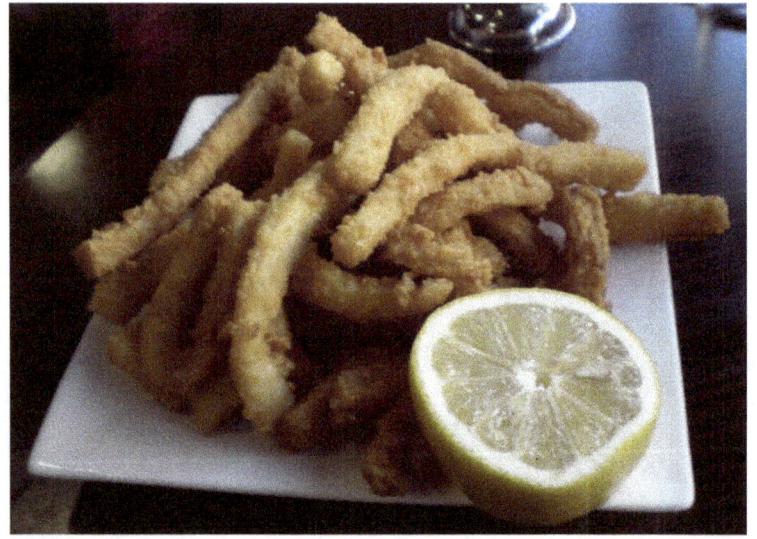

Preparation Time: 5 minutes

Cooking Time: 12 minutes

Servings: 4

Ingredients:

- 16 rabas
- 1 egg
- Breadcrumbs

- Salt, pepper, sweet paprika

Directions:

1. Put the rabas in the Air Fryer to boil for 2 minutes.
2. Remove and dry well. Beat the egg and season to taste. You can put salt, pepper and sweet paprika. Place in the egg.
3. Bread with breadcrumbs. Place in sticks.
4. Air fry for 10 minutes at 360°F

Nutrition:

Calories 356

Fat 18g

Carbs 5 g

Protein 34g

Honey Glazed Salmon

Preparation Time: 10 minutes

Cooking Time: 8 minutes

Servings: 2

Ingredients:

- 2 (6 oz.) salmon fillets
- Salt, as required
- 2 tbsp. honey

Directions:

1. Sprinkle the salmon fillets with salt and then, coat with honey.
2. Preheat at 355°F.
3. Arrange the salmon fillets in greased Air Fryer basket and insert in the Air Fryer. Cook for 8 minutes. Serve hot.

Nutrition:

Calories 289

Fat 10.5g

Carbs 17.3g

Protein 33.1g

Sweet & Sour Glazed Salmon

Preparation Time: 12 minutes

Cooking Time: 20 minutes

Servings: 2

Ingredients:

- 1/3 cup soy sauce
- 1/3 cup honey
- 3 tsp.s rice wine vinegar
- 1 tsp. water
- 4 (3½-oz.) salmon fillets

Directions:

1. Mix the soy sauce, honey, vinegar, and water together in a bowl.
2. In another small bowl, reserve about half of the mixture.
3. Add salmon fillets in the remaining mixture and coat well.
4. Cover the bowl and refrigerate to marinate for about 2 hours.

5. Preheat at 355°F.
6. Arrange the salmon fillets in greased Air Fryer basket and insert in the Air Fryer. Cook for 12 minutes
7. Flip the salmon fillets once halfway through and coat with the reserved marinade after every 3 minutes.
8. Serve hot.

Nutrition:

Calories 462

Fat 12.3g

Carbs 49.8g

Protein 41.3g

Ranch Tilapia

Preparation Time: 15 minutes

Cooking Time: 13 minutes

Servings: 4

Ingredients:

- ¾ cup cornflakes, crushed
- 1 (1-oz.) packet dry ranch-style dressing mix
- 2½ tbsp. vegetable oil
- 2 eggs
- 4 (6-oz.) tilapia fillets

Directions:

1. In a shallow bowl, beat the eggs.
2. In another bowl, add the cornflakes, ranch dressing, and oil and mix until a crumbly mixture form.
3. Dip the fish fillets into egg and then, coat with the bread crumbs mixture.
4. Preheat at 356°F.

5. Arrange the tilapia fillets in greased Air Fryer basket and insert in the Air Fryer. Cook for 13 minutes. Serve hot.

Nutrition:

Calories 267

Fat 12.2g

Carbs 5.1g

Protein 34.9g

Breaded Flounder

Preparation Time: 15 minutes

Cooking Time: 12 minutes

Servings: 3

Ingredients:

- 1 egg
- 1 cup dry breadcrumbs
- ¼ cup vegetable oil
- 3 (6-oz.) flounder fillets
- 1 lemon, sliced

Directions:

1. In a shallow bowl, beat the egg
2. In another bowl, add the breadcrumbs and oil and mix until a crumbly mixture is formed.
3. Dip flounder fillets into the beaten egg and then coat with the breadcrumb mixture.
4. Preheat at 355°F.

5. Arrange the flounder fillets in greased Air Fryer basket and insert in the Air Fryer. Cook for 12 minutes
6. Plate with lemon slices and serve hot.

Nutrition:

Calories 524

Fat 24.2g

Carbs 26.5g

Protein 47.8g

Simple Haddock

Preparation Time: 15 minutes

Cooking Time: 8 minutes

Servings: 2

Ingredients:

- 2 (6-oz.) haddock fillets
- 1 tbsp. olive oil
- Salt and ground black pepper, as required

Directions:

1. Coat the fish fillets with oil and then, sprinkle with salt and black pepper.
2. Preheat at 355°F.
3. Arrange the haddock fillets in greased Air Fryer basket and insert in the Air Fryer. Cook for 8 minutes. Serve hot.

Nutrition:

Calories 251

Fat 8.6g

Saturated Fat 1.3g

Carbs 0g

Protein 41.2g

Breaded Hake

Preparation Time: 15 minutes

Cooking Time: 12 minutes

Servings: 4

Ingredients:

- 1 egg
- 4 oz. breadcrumbs
- 2 tbsp. vegetable oil
- 4 (6-oz.) hake fillets
- 1 lemon, cut into wedges

Directions:

1. In a shallow bowl, whisk the egg.
2. In another bowl, add the breadcrumbs, and oil and mix until a crumbly mixture forms.
3. Dip fish fillets into the egg and then, coat with the bread crumbs mixture.
4. Preheat at 350°F.

5. Arrange the hake fillets in greased Air Fryer basket and insert in the Air Fryer. Cook for 12 minutes. Serve hot.

Nutrition:

Calories 297

Fat 10.6g

Carbs 22g

Protein 29.2g

Sesame Seeds Coated Tuna

Preparation Time: 15 minutes

Cooking Time: 6 minutes

Servings: 2

Ingredients:

- 1 egg white
- ¼ cup white sesame seeds
- 1 tbsp. black sesame seeds
- Salt and ground black pepper, as required
- 2 (6-oz.) tuna steaks

Directions:

1. In a bowl, beat the egg white.
2. In another bowl, mix together the sesame seeds, salt, and black pepper.
3. Dip the tuna steaks into the egg white and then coat with the sesame seeds mixture.

4. Preheat at 355°F. Arrange the tuna steak fillets in greased Air Fryer basket and insert in the Air Fryer. Cook for 8 minutes
5. Flip the tuna steaks once halfway through. Serve hot.

Nutrition:

Calories 450

Fat 21.9g

Carbs 5.4g

Protein 56.7g

Air-Fried Seafood

Preparation Time: 10 minutes

Cooking Time: 10 minutes

Servings: 4

Ingredients:

- 1 lb. fresh scallops, mussels, fish fillets, prawns, shrimp
- 2 eggs, lightly beaten
- Salt and black pepper
- 1 cup breadcrumbs mixed with the zest of 1 lemon
- Cooking spray

Directions:

1. Clean the seafood as needed.
2. Dip each piece into the egg and season with salt and pepper.
3. Coat in the crumbs and spray with oil.

4. Arrange into the Air Fryer and cook for 6 minutes at 400°F turning once halfway through. Serve and Enjoy!

Nutrition:

Calories 133

Protein 17.4g

Fat 3.1g

Carbs 8.2g

Fish with Chips

Preparation Time: 5 minutes

Cooking Time: 20 minutes

Servings: 2

Ingredients:

- 1 cod fillet (6 oz.)
- 3 cups salt
- 3 cups vinegar-flavored kettle cooked chips
- ¼ cup buttermilk
- salt and pepper to taste

Directions:

1. Mix to combine the buttermilk, pepper, and salt in a bowl. Put the cod and leave to soak for 5 minutes
2. Put the chips in a food processor and process until crushed. Transfer to a shallow bowl. Coat the fillet with the crushed chips.

3. Put the coated fillet in the air frying basket. Cook for 12 minutes at 400°F. Serve and Enjoy!

Nutrition:

Calories 646

Fat 33g

Protein 41g

Carbs 48g

Crumbly Fishcakes

Preparation Time: 5 minutes

Cooking Time: 10 minutes

Servings: 4

Ingredients:

- 8 oz. salmon, cooked
- 1 ½ oz. potatoes, mashed
- A handful of parsley, chopped
- Zest of 1 lemon
- 1 ¾ oz. plain flour

Directions:

1. Carefully flakes the salmon. In a bowl, mix flaked salmon, zest, capers, dill, and mashed potatoes.
2. From small cakes using the mixture and dust the cakes with flour; refrigerate for 60 minutes.
3. Preheat your Air Fryer to 350°F. and cook the cakes for 7 minutes. Serve chilled.

Nutrition:

Calories 210

Protein 10g

Fat 7g

Carbs 25g

Bacon Wrapped Shrimp

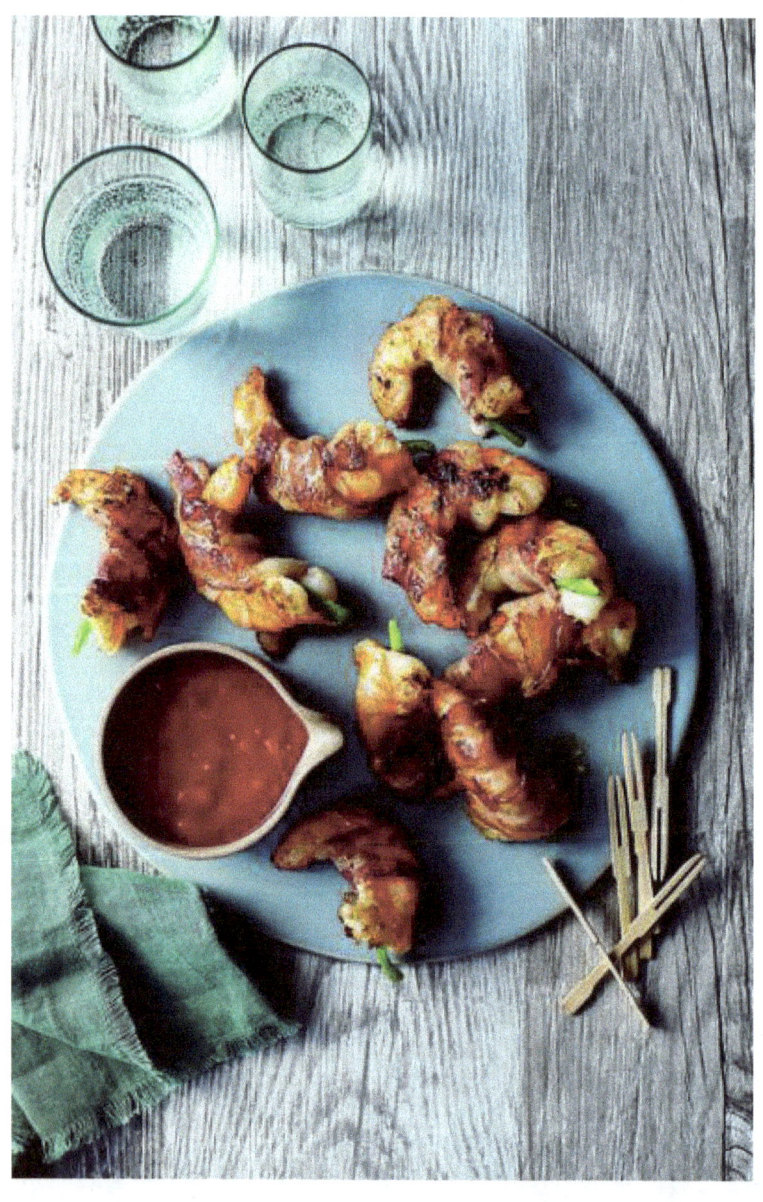

Preparation Time: 10 minutes

Cooking Time: 20 minutes

Servings: 4

Ingredients:

- 16 thin slices of bacon
- 16 pieces of tiger shrimp (peeled and deveined)

Directions:

1. With a slice of bacon, wrap each shrimp. Put all the finished pieces in tray and chill for 20 minutes.
2. Arrange the bacon-wrapped shrimp in the air frying basket. Cook for 7 minutes at 390°F. Transfer to a plate lined with paper towels to drain before serving.

Nutrition:

Calories 436

Protein 32g

Fat 41.01g

Carbs 0.8g

Crab Legs

Preparation Time: 10 minutes

Cooking Time: 10 minutes

Servings: 4

Ingredients:

- 3 lb. crab legs
- ¼ cup salted butter, melted and divided
- ½ lemon, juiced
- ¼ tsp. garlic powder

Directions:

1. In a bowl, toss the crab legs and two tbsp. of the melted butter together. Place the crab legs in the basket of the fryer.
2. Cook at 400°F for fifteen minutes, giving the basket a good shake halfway through.
3. Combine the remaining butter with the lemon juice and garlic powder.

4. Crack open the cooked crab legs and remove the meat. Serve with the butter dip on the side, and enjoy!

Nutrition:

Calories 272

Fat 19g

Carbs 18g

Protein 12g

Fish Sticks

Preparation Time: 5 minutes

Cooking Time: 10 minutes

Servings: 4

Ingredients:

- 1 lb. whitefish
- 2 tbsp. Dijon mustard
- ¼ cup mayonnaise
- 1 ½ cup pork rinds, finely ground
- ¾ tsp. Cajun seasoning

Directions:

1. Place the fish on a tissue to dry it off, then cut it up into slices about two inches thick.
2. In one bowl, combine the mustard and mayonnaise, and in another, the Cajun seasoning and pork rinds.

3. Coat the fish firstly in the mayo-mustard mixture, then in the Cajun-pork rind mixture. Give each slice a shake to remove any surplus. Then place the fish sticks in the basket of the air flyer.
4. Cook at 400°F for five minutes. Turn the fish sticks over and cook for another five minutes on the other side.
5. Serve warm with a dipping sauce of your choosing and enjoy.

Nutrition:

Calories 212

Fat 12g

Carbs 14g

Protein 8g

Crusty Pesto Salmon

Preparation Time: 5 minutes

Cooking Time: 10 minutes

Servings: 2

Ingredients:

- ¼ cup almonds, roughly chopped
- ¼ cup pesto
- 2 x 4-oz. salmon fillets
- 2 tbsp. unsalted butter, melted

Directions:

1. Mix the almonds and pesto together.
2. Place the salmon fillets in a round baking dish, roughly six inches in diameter.
3. Brush the fillets with butter, followed by the pesto mixture, ensuring to coat both the top and bottom. Put the baking dish inside the fryer.
4. Cook for twelve minutes at 390°F.

5. The salmon is ready when it flakes easily when prodded with a fork. Serve warm.

Nutrition:

Calories 354

Fat 21g

Carbs 23g

Protein 19g

Salmon Patties

Preparation Time: 5 minutes

Cooking Time: 10 minutes

Servings: 4

Ingredients:

- 1 tsp. chili powder
- 2 tbsp. full-fat mayonnaise
- ¼ cup ground pork rinds
- 2 x 5-oz. pouches of cooked pink salmon
- 1 egg

Directions:

1. Stir everything together to prepare the patty mixture. If the mixture is dry or falling apart, add in more pork rinds as necessary.
2. Take equal-sized amounts of the mixture to form four patties, before placing the patties in the basket of your Air Fryer.

3. Cook at 400°F for eight minutes.
4. Halfway through cooking, flip the patties over. Once they are crispy, serve with the toppings of your choice and enjoy.

Nutrition:

Calories 325

Fat 21g

Carbs 18g

Protein 29g

Buttery Cod

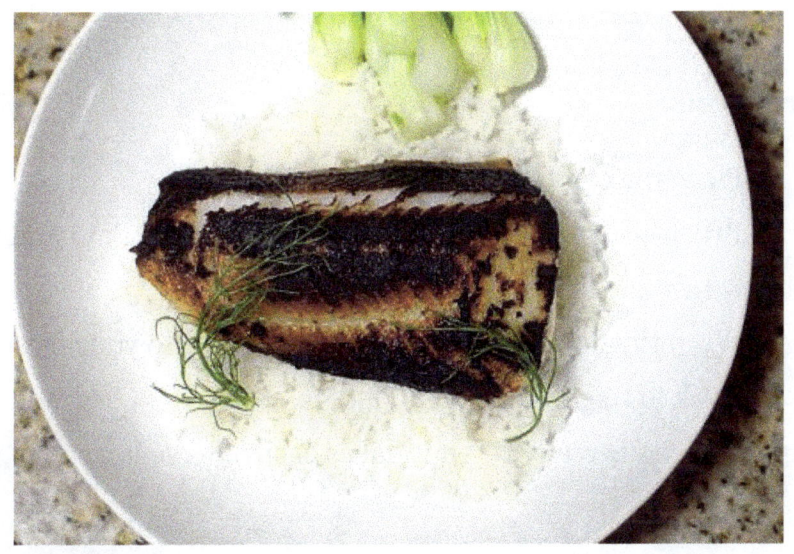

Preparation Time: 5 minutes

Cooking Time: 10 minutes

Servings: 4

Ingredients:

- 2 x 4-oz. cod fillets
- 2 tbsp. salted butter, melted

- 1 tsp. Old Bay seasoning
- ½ medium lemon, sliced

Directions:

1. Place the cod fillets in a dish.
2. Brush with melted butter, season with Old Bay, and top with some lemon slices.
3. Wrap the fish in aluminum foil and put into your fryer.
4. Cook for eight minutes at 350°F.
5. The cod is ready when it flakes easily. Serve hot.

Nutrition:

Calories 354

Fat 21g

Carbs 23g

Protein 19g

Sesame Tuna Steak

Preparation Time: 5 minutes

Cooking Time: 10 minutes

Servings: 4

Ingredients:

- 1 tbsp. coconut oil, melted
- 2 x 6-oz. tuna steaks
- ½ tsp. garlic powder
- 2 tsp. black sesame seeds
- 2 tsp. white sesame seeds

Directions:

1. Apply the coconut oil to the tuna steaks with a brunch, then season with garlic powder.
2. Combine the black and white sesame seeds. Embed them in the tuna steaks, covering the fish all over. Place the tuna into your Air Fryer.

3. Cook for eight minutes at 400°F, turning the fish halfway through.
4. The tuna steaks are ready when they have reached a temperature of 145°F. Serve straight away.

Nutrition:

Calories 343

Fat 11g

Carbs 27g

Protein 25g

Lemon Garlic Shrimp

Preparation Time: 5 minutes

Cooking Time: 10 minutes

Servings: 4

Ingredients:

- 1 medium lemon
- ½ lb. medium shrimp, shelled and deveined
- ½ tsp. Old Bay seasoning
- 2 tbsp. unsalted butter, melted
- ½ tsp. minced garlic

Directions:

1. Grate the lemon rind into a bowl. Cut the lemon in half then juice it over the same bowl. Toss in the shrimp, Old Bay, and butter, mixing everything to make sure the shrimp is completely covered.
2. Transfer to a round baking dish roughly six inches wide, then place this dish in your Air Fryer.

3. Cook at 400°F for six minutes. The shrimp is ready when it becomes a bright pink color.
4. Serve hot, drizzling any leftover sauce over the shrimp.

Nutrition:

Calories 374

Fat 14g

Carbs 18g

Protein 21g

Foil Packet Salmon

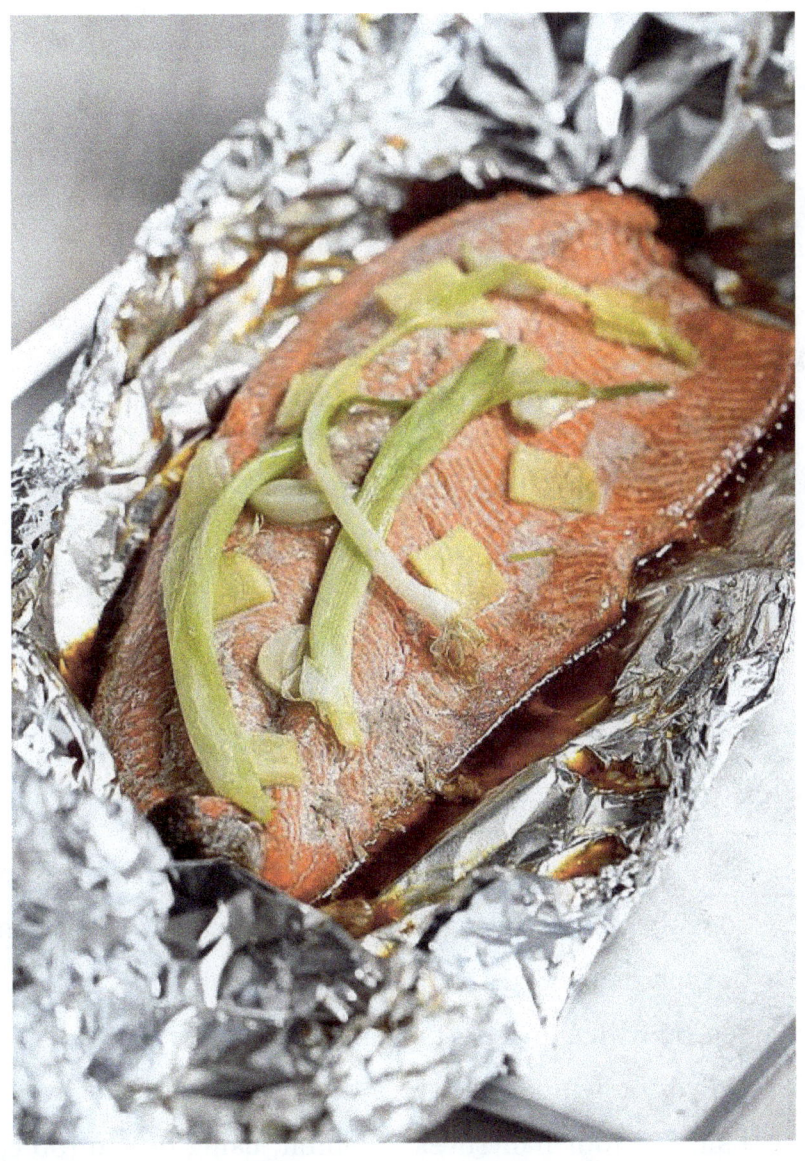

Preparation Time: 5 minutes

Cooking Time: 10 minutes

Servings: 4

Ingredients:

- 2 x 4-oz. skinless salmon fillets
- 2 tbsp. unsalted butter, melted
- ½ tsp. garlic powder
- 1 medium lemon
- ½ tsp. dried dill

Directions:

1. Take a sheet of foil and cut into two squares measuring roughly 5" x 5". Lay each of the salmon fillets at the center of each piece. Brush both fillets with a tbsp. of bullet and season with a quarter-tsp. of garlic powder.
2. Halve the lemon and grate the skin of one half over the fish. Cut four half-slices of lemon, using two to top each fillet. Season each fillet with a quarter-tsp. of dill.

3. Fold the tops and sides of the aluminum foil over the fish to create a kind of packet. Place each one in the fryer.
4. Cook for twelve minutes at 400°F.
5. The salmon is ready when it flakes easily. Serve hot.

Nutrition:

Calories 365

Fat 16g

Carbs 18g

Protein 23g

Foil Packet Lobster Tail

Preparation Time: 5 minutes

Cooking Time: 10 minutes

Servings: 4

Ingredients:

- 2 x 6-oz. lobster tail halves
- 2 tbsp. salted butter, melted
- ½ medium lemon, juiced
- ½ tsp. Old Bay seasoning
- 1 tsp. dried parsley

Directions:

1. Lay each lobster on a sheet of aluminum foil. Pour a light drizzle of melted butter and lemon juice over each one, and season with Old Bay.
2. Fold down the sides and ends of the foil to seal the lobster. Place each one in the fryer.
3. Cook at 375°F for twelve minutes.

4. Just before serving, top the lobster with dried parsley.

Nutrition:

Calories 369

Fat 19g

Carbs 25g

Protein 28g

Avocado Shrimp

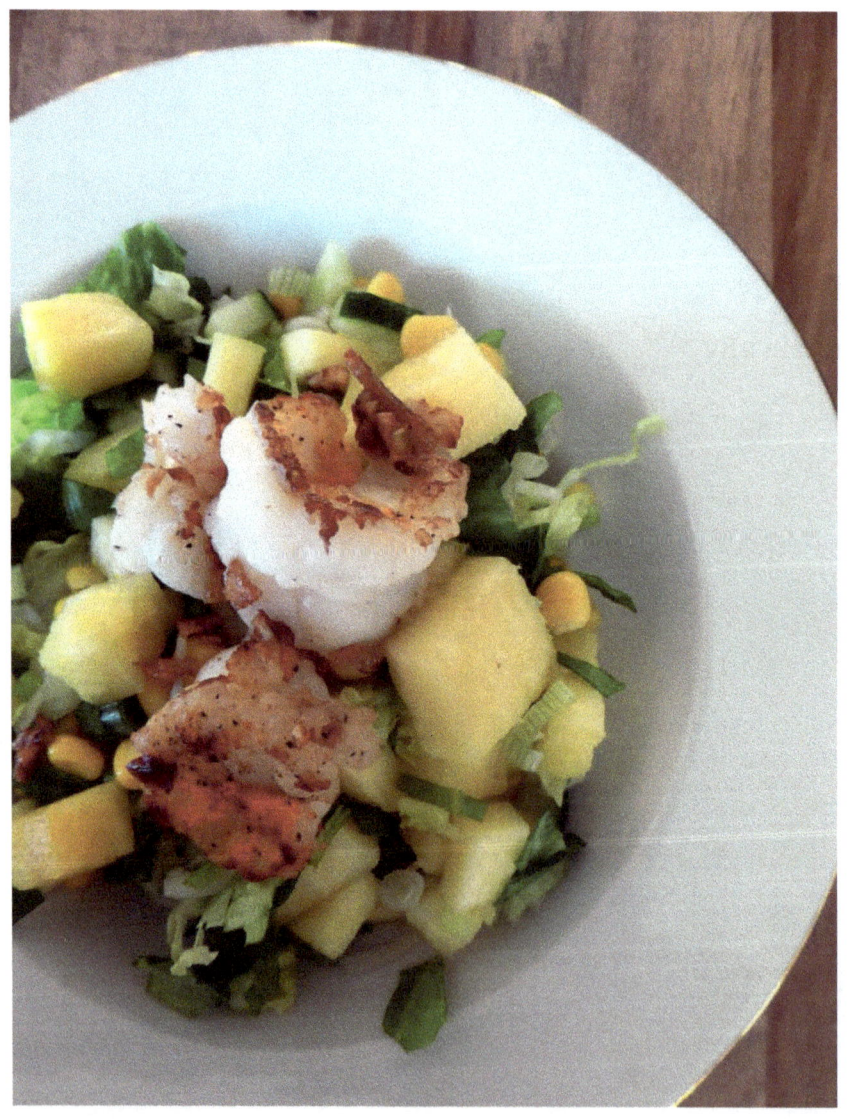

Preparation Time: 5 minutes

Cooking Time: 10 minutes

Servings: 4

Ingredients:

- ½ cup onion, chopped
- 2 lb. shrimp
- 1 tbsp. seasoned salt
- 1 avocado
- ½ cup pecans, chopped

Directions:

1. Pre-heat the fryer at 400°F.
2. Put the chopped onion in the basket of the fryer and spritz with some cooking spray. Leave to cook for five minutes.
3. Add the shrimp and set the timer for a further five minutes. Sprinkle with some seasoned salt, then allow to cook for an additional five minutes.
4. During these last five minutes, halve your avocado and remove the pit. Cube each half, then scoop out the flesh.

5. Take care when removing the shrimp from the fryer. Place it on a dish and top with the avocado and the chopped pecans.

Nutrition:

Calories 384

Fat 24g

Carbs 13g

Protein 39g

Citrusy Branzini on the Grill

Preparation Time: 5 minutes

Cooking Time: 15 minutes

Servings: 4

Ingredients:

- 4 branzini fillets
- Salt and pepper to taste
- 2 lemons, juice freshly squeezed
- 2 oranges, juice freshly squeezed

Directions:

1. Place all ingredients in a Ziploc bag. Keep it in the fridge for 2 hours.
2. Preheat the Air Fryer at 390°F. Place the grill pan attachment in the Air Fryer.
3. Place the fish on the grill pan and cook for 15 minutes until the fish is flaky.

Nutrition:

Calories 318

Fat 15.6g

Carbs 20.8g

Protein 23.5g

Cajun-Seasoned Lemon Salmon

Preparation Time: 5 minutes

Cooking Time: 10 minutes

Servings: 4

Ingredients:

- 1 salmon fillet
- 1 tsp. Cajun seasoning
- lemon wedges, for serving
- 1 tsp. liquid stevia
- ½ lemon, juiced

Directions:

1. Preheat your Air Fryer to 350°F. Combine lemon juice and liquid stevia and coat salmon with this mixture. Sprinkle Cajun seasoning all over salmon. Place salmon on parchment paper in Air Fryer and cook for 7-minutes. Serve with lemon wedges.

Nutrition:

Calories 287

Fat 9.3g

Carbs 8.4g

Protein 15.3g

Grilled Salmon Fillets

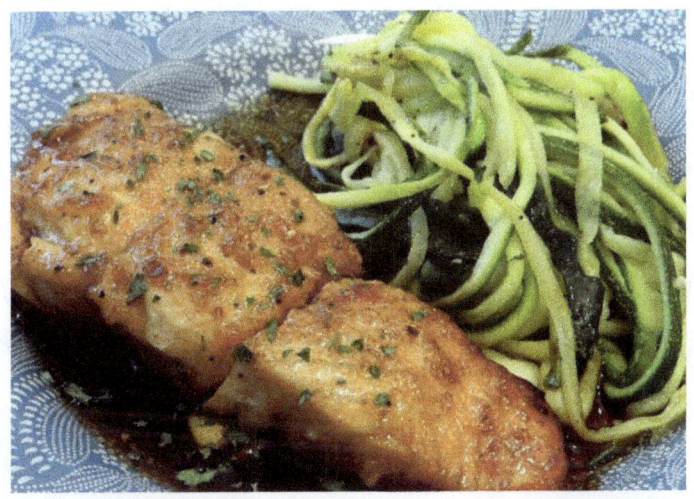

Preparation Time: 5 minutes

Cooking Time: 10 minutes

Servings: 4

Ingredients:

- salmon fillets
- tbsp. olive oil
- 1/3 cup of light soy sauce

- 1/3 cup of water
- Salt and black pepper to taste

Directions:

Season salmon fillets with salt and pepper. Mix what's left of the ingredients in a bowl. Allow the salmon fillets to marinate in mixture for 2-hours. Preheat your Air Fryer to 355°F for 5-minutes. Drain salmon fillets and air fry for 8-minutes.

Nutrition:

Calories 302

Fat 8.6g

Carbs 7.3g

Protein 15.3g

Cheesy Breaded Salmon

Preparation Time: 5 minutes

Cooking Time: 20 minutes

Servings: 4

Ingredients:

- cups breadcrumbs
- salmon fillets
- eggs, beaten
- 1 cup Swiss cheese, shredded

Directions:

Preheat your Air Fryer to 390°F. Dip each salmon filet into eggs. Top with Swiss cheese. Dip into breadcrumbs, coating entire fish. Put into an oven-safe dish and cook for 20-minutes.

Nutrition:

Calories 296

Fat 9.2g

Carbs 8.7g

Protein 15.2g

Coconut Crusted Shrimp

Preparation Time: 15 minutes

Cooking Time: 40 minutes

Servings: 4

Ingredients:

- oz. coconut milk
- ½ cup sweetened coconut, shredded
- ½ cup panko breadcrumbs
- 1-lb. large shrimp, peeled and deveined
- Salt and black pepper, to taste

Directions:

2. Preheat the Air Fryer to 350°F and grease an Air Fryer basket.
3. Place the coconut milk in a shallow bowl.
4. Mix coconut, breadcrumbs, salt, and black pepper in another bowl.

5. Dip each shrimp into coconut milk and finally, dredge in the coconut mixture.
6. Arrange half of the shrimps into the Air Fryer basket and cook for about 20 minutes.
7. Dish out the shrimps onto serving plates and repeat with the remaining mixture to serve.

Nutrition:

Calories 408

Fats: 23.7g

Carbs 11.7g

Proteins: 31g,

Rice Flour Coated Shrimp

Preparation Time: 20 minutes

Cooking Time: 20 minutes

Servings: 3

Ingredients:

- tbsp. rice flour
- 1-lb. shrimp, peeled and deveined
- tbsp. olive oil
- 1 tsp. powdered sugar
- Salt and black pepper, as required

Directions:

1. Preheat the Air Fryer to 325°F and grease an Air Fryer basket.
2. Mix rice flour, olive oil, sugar, salt, and black pepper in a bowl.
3. Stir in the shrimp and transfer half of the shrimp to the Air Fryer basket.

4. Cook for about 10 minutes, flipping once in between.
5. Dish out the mixture onto serving plates and repeat with the remaining mixture.

Nutrition:

Calories 299

Fat 12g

Carbs 11.1g

Protein 35g

www.ingramcontent.com/pod-product-compliance
Lightning Source LLC
Chambersburg PA
CBHW071107030426
42336CB00013BA/1986